Bhakti and Karma Yoga

–

The Science of Devotion
and
Liberation Through Action

Yogani

From The AYP Enlightenment Series

AYP Publishing

For ordering information go to:

www.advancedyogapractices.com

Library of Congress Control Number: 2008901443

Published simultaneously in:

Nashville, Tennessee, U.S.A.
and
London, England, U.K.

This title is also available in eBook format – ISBN 978-0-9800522-6-8
(For Adobe Reader)

ISBN 978-0-9800522-4-4 (Paperback)

"I have lived on the lip of insanity, wanting
to know reasons, knocking on a door.
It opens.
I have been knocking from the inside!"

Jelaluddin Rumi – 13th Century Sufi Mystic

Introduction

Desire is the root of all action, and action is what produces change in human life, for good or ill. Therefore, informing our desires with a chosen high ideal and implementing our intentions accordingly in spiritual practices and daily activity will have a profound influence on many outcomes in our life.

Bhakti and Karma Yoga covers the systematic application of the essential principles of desire and devotion to aid us in achieving our goals and spiritual aspirations. Through inspired action we can transform our life experience to one of ecstatic bliss. In combination with an effective daily routine of yoga practices, the principles of bhakti and karma yoga elevate the relationship of our desires and actions to divine expression, greatly hastening our progress toward enlightenment.

The AYP Enlightenment Series is an endeavor to present the most effective methods of spiritual practice in a series of easy-to-read books that anyone can use to gain practical results immediately and over the long term. Since its beginnings in 2003, *Advanced Yoga Practices (AYP)* has been an experiment to see just how much can be conveyed in writing, with much more detail provided on practices than in the spiritual writings of the past.

Can books provide us the specific means necessary to tread the path to enlightenment, or do we have to surrender at the feet of a *guru* to find our salvation? Well, clearly we must surrender to something, even if it is to our own innate potential to live a freer and happier life. If we are able to do that, and maintain regular practice, then books like this one can come alive and instruct us in the ways of human spiritual transformation. If the reader is ready and the book is worthy, amazing things can happen.

While one person's name is given as the author of this book, it is actually a distillation of the efforts of thousands of practitioners over thousands of years. This is one person's attempt to simplify and make practical the spiritual methods that many have demonstrated throughout history. All who have gone before have my deepest gratitude, as do the many I am privileged to be in touch with in the present who continue to practice with dedication and good results.

I hope you will find this book to be a useful resource as you travel along your chosen path.

Practice wisely, and enjoy!

Table of Contents

Chapter 1 – Desire and Action

Desire is fundamental to our existence. But desire does not stand alone. For what is a desire if it is not acted upon? Nothing but an unresolved hankering. Indeed, desire without action is like a driver without a vehicle. And action without a clear desire to guide it is like a machine running hither and yon without rhyme or reason.

There has sometimes been criticism of the presence of desire on the spiritual path, even to the point of calling for the end of desire. This is because desire does not always lead to results that may be considered positive. Negative desires can lead to negative results when acted upon, while positive desires will most often lead to positive results. The laws we have in society, while they may seem to be about limiting harmful actions, are really about limiting the effects of negative desires.

Because the precautions of the law are necessary in society, does this mean that all desires are bad? Obviously not. If we have a positive intent to limit the effect of negative desires, then the final outcome will inevitably be positive. This is the classic struggle of "good over evil." It revolves around our desires, and the actions they inspire.

To say that all desires are bad is to say that all human endeavor is bad, and that we should not do anything. It is a foolish proposition. Much better to face things as they are and see how we can make something good out of it, something useful. The dynamics of desire and action offer endless possibilities for good, including our ultimate enlightenment. It is a journey of divine attraction and love for our own highest ideal, culminating in the transformation of experience in all aspects of our everyday living. This has profound implications for us, and for everyone around us. By changing ourselves, we can change the world!

But before we talk about enlightenment and how desire and action can open our life up to it, let's examine how the basic principles of desire and action relate to our everyday life. Then we will look deeper and see how these same principles can take us far beyond the ordinary to the extraordinary, even as we continue to live a normal life much as we did before.

Everyone wants something. We are each born with inclinations – the seeds that germinate within us to become our desires in life, influenced by the environment we grow up in.

There is another influence on the shape and direction our desires may take, and that is the cycle of our desire and resulting action, leading to more desire and action, in kind. It is the natural cycle of desires and actions leading to more and more. Once we are in this cycle, action leads to desire just as desire leads to action. Round and round it goes, and we may lose track of which came first, the desire or the action. It is the proverbial question: "Which came first, the chicken or the egg?"

As we all know, this endless cycle of desires and actions can lead to what seems to be a treadmill in life. Or it can lead to remarkable achievements if we have an underlying vision, or central theme, guiding our desires and actions. With a clear vision in place, the endless cycle of desire and action can be used with great effectiveness. This is the key to all achievements by successful people, whether it be the local shopkeeper, or one who is able to enhance the quality of life for all of humanity. It is a clear vision of possibilities that can lift desire and action to a higher purpose, and there is no limit in this. It is limited only by our imagination.

The relationship between a vision and the mechanics of desire and action is well known by those who strive to great achievements, and we can see it in action everywhere around us. It can be seen as *cause and effect*, which puts it into the realm of science, whereby the application of known principles will produce predictable results:

Vision + Desire + Action = Achievement

...with *persistence and consistency* being underlying qualities found in all of the elements on the left side of the equation.

All that we accomplish in life has a vision behind it, though we may not recognize a vision because it has become automatic – programmed within our subconscious mind. The small things we accomplish have small visions behind them, like getting up in the morning, getting dressed and going out. The larger things we accomplish have larger visions behind them, like caring for our family and pursuing our career. The greater our vision, the greater the possibilities for what we can accomplish in this life.

Visions may be ingrained in us and may seem to be fixed, sometimes to our disadvantage. But visions can be changed, and new and greater ones can be created if we are willing to put in the time and effort to reprogram our inner habits. Desire is always seeking more, and that more is found in the form of an expanded vision, which will focus desire like a laser beam, yielding miraculous results. There are powerful tools available to aid in this, which we will be discussing in this book.

If we have a clear vision of what we want, and are willing to act on it every day for as long as it takes to see our vision fulfilled, then there is no limit to what we can accomplish. When desire has been raised to this level of constancy in a particular vision, then it is called *devotion*. In the language of Yoga, this is called *Bhakti*. Those who live their life in constant devotion to their vision find support coming from all sides, and are able to overcome seemingly insurmountable obstacles.

Handicaps are not able to hold back a person who persistently acts on desires that are rooted in a clear vision. In fact, handicaps can provide an advantage to the person persistently acting on their vision, because handicaps are clear obstructions which must be overcome on the way to fulfillment. Handicaps provide constant reminders that there is more to be done.

Just so, a poor man with a strong desire to become rich has an advantage over a rich man who does not have a vision for his life. The obstacles the poor man must overcome are milestones on the way to fulfillment of his vision. Likewise, if a rich man wishes to grow, he too must overcome obstacles on the way to a truth of greater significance than his current bank account. Is that greater truth a bigger bank account? It might be. It all depends on the vision that is chosen.

In the long run, the visionary choices we make that inform our unending cycles of desire-action-desire-action will determine the degree of happiness and fulfillment we find in life. Our vision, our desire and our actions will have consequences. In spiritual language, the actions we undertake and their consequences are summed up in the phrase, "As you sow, so shall you reap." This is what we mean by *Karma*. As we become increasingly sensitive to the results of our actions, our vision of life, our desires, and our actions will be affected accordingly.

The principles of vision, desire and action operate the same in spiritual life as they do in material life. In fact, these are at the core of spiritual life, just as they are at the core of anything we may undertake in this world. If we are looking for fulfillment that reaches beyond the limitations of our material world, even while we are still living fully in it, then sooner or later we will come to consider the spiritual dimension. It is a natural thing, because everyone is wired inside for a greater destiny than may meet the eye, much greater than we may have imagined so far.

It is not a coincidence that desire for and devotion to a higher vision of truth is at the core of every religion in the world. It is the inherent longing for this in human beings that has created the religions, and not the other way around. In fact, the realization of our innate human spiritual potential can occur entirely without the trappings of religion, and often does. Religion is there to remind us of what we already are in seed form. Once we have sensed our potential, it is up to us to make the necessary choices to move forward according to our own vision, rather than anyone else's. The institutions will call us to their fold, but the real fold is in us. It is an inner opening into a fullness that is beyond worldly considerations, even though worldly considerations will go on, illuminated from within. We are fortunate to be living in a time when this kind of inner renaissance is happening at an ever-increasing rate. It is through the rise of individual enlightenment on a mass scale that our society is gradually being transformed. It is a choice that we are in a much better position to make than in centuries past, because of both inner and outer events. We are all interconnected in that. The rise of spiritual desire goes far beyond the individual. It is a global phenomenon that we all have a stake in.

On the inside, the obstructions to the natural divine flow in the human neurobiology are becoming less, and the possibilities are thus becoming clearer to everyone. Spiritual experiences that seemed impossible not long ago are becoming common among many. What before may have been a faint inspiration of our divine possibilities is now becoming a loud inner trumpet that can be easily heard. It is inspiration that leads to realization. A core component of this inner awakening is ever-increasing spiritual desire. The energy rising in us now is so great that it cries out to be acted upon. It is vision, desire and a call to action, all in one. We are each experiencing it in our own way.

On the outside, the availability of spiritual knowledge is increasing, and the vehicles for its delivery are becoming more efficient and readily accessible, thanks to modern communications and more practical scientific approaches. We are in the midst of a spiritual knowledge revolution. While there can be some confusion in this, there is also the opportunity for systematic integrations and applications of knowledge in ways that were not possible in the past. This is particularly true of powerful spiritual practices that have long been held in secret in fragments around the world. Now, for the first time, the secrets are dissolving and the fragments are being joined and applied in ways that serve the need of our time. Causes and effects in spiritual practice are being examined systematically much more so than in the past, and adjustments are occurring to optimize results, lifting the field of spiritual practice to the level of real science. So it is a new era of spiritual knowledge, practice and experience. This is having a profound effect on spiritual seekers everywhere, and on their actions flowing from the accelerating surge of spiritual desire coming from within.

Together, increasing internal spiritual desire and increasing external resources for spiritual knowledge, are producing a dynamic that has not been seen in human history. Never before has it been so easy to fulfill the promise of salvation found in the ancient scriptures, summed up in the Christian maxim:

"Seek and you will find. Knock and the door will open."

Many are eagerly knocking, and many doors are opening ... being opened from the inside!

This remarkable phenomenon is not limited by culture or religion, and is, in fact, occurring in millions of people living in all of the world's cultures and religions. Change is in the air…

Now let's look at the specifics of how the underlying principles of vision, desire and action function on our spiritual path, and what we can do to enhance the process for maximum results.

Chapter 2 – Bhakti Yoga

The classical definition of bhakti yoga is *union through devotion*. By devotion, we mean the continuous flow of desire in accordance with a vision. We can also call the vision an *ideal*, and it is chosen by each of us in a very individual and personal way.

Bhakti is the primary engine of all spiritual progress, and of all spiritual practices we may undertake to enhance our spiritual progress. It is our longing that must be stirring before we can take the steps necessary to grow. Longing is an emotion, a need. We don't even have to know what it is we are needing. The feeling is enough to make things happen, assuming we are willing to act. The desire comes first. Then comes action. And from action we see more that we can experience and know, and our longing is further stimulated by that.

The simple process just described is an organic one, and is at the heart of every spiritual journey and of every religion. It is human longing for answers about our ultimate purpose and destiny that drives the mechanisms of spiritual experience and realization everywhere on the earth. And so too does human longing for truth drive the religions that serve this great purpose to the extent they are able to transcend their political agendas and institutional limitations. It is not so complicated.

While we may have been taught that our salvation is in the hands of this or that god or religious institution, our salvation is in our own hands according to our own longing and willingness to act upon it. <u>The human nervous system is the center of all spiritual progress, not any authority outside us.</u> This isn't to say we will not be devoted to the deity or ideal we have known since childhood, or to any other we may be drawn to in our life. There are innumerable sources of spiritual inspiration and energy in the world. But it is we who open the valve for that energy to flow into our life. When we are ready, the spiritual energy will flow. When the valve is continuously open by our own desire and action, then we will find ourselves living in a state of grace. Ongoing bhakti and grace are two sides of the same coin.

We may give all that we have and do to our god or our chosen ideal. It is our own devotion that creates the freedom and happiness we are living. That is grace. It is a fascinating dynamic, giving credence to the phrase, "The more we give, the more we receive."

It is in our own hands. But only to the extent we are ready. Fortunately, it is not all or nothing. We can inch our way into the increasingly powerful dynamic of bhakti. Contrary to what we may have been taught, there are no absolutes in the field of devotion. We can begin with the simplest of inquires, like, "Who am I" and "What am I doing here?"

If we ask with longing, the answers will begin to come, and we can move forward from there. This is the wonder of bhakti. It is very systematic and can function with the effective use of any emotion we may be experiencing here and now. The results of applied bhakti are predictable and repeatable, leading us to call bhakti *the science of devotion.*

The journey of bhakti and of human spiritual transformation is a continuum, not an instant event. It is occurring right here, right now, and our realization of truth can evolve naturally within the life we are living. No need to run off to the mountain top, or trade in our family and career for robes and exotic gurus. These veneers are insignificant in relation to a longing heart expressing itself in ordinary life. Enlightenment is not about place. It is about desire and its expression in effective spiritual practices, and how that overflows into the conduct of our daily life.

Bhakti – Up Close and Personal

Traditionally, bhakti is considered to be *love of God*, which usually places it in the realm of religion. This well and good, but there is another side of bhakti that is not necessarily religious. Bhakti may also be regarded as *spiritual* without any religious affiliation.

There are many forms of bhakti, as many as there are *ishtas* (chosen ideals) and attributes that we can imagine. Unlimited! Here, we will not get into well-known traditional expressions of bhakti very much. It is the province of the religions. For those who love to worship in their religious tradition, that is very good. For those who are not inclined that way, it is not the end of the world. Yoga and spiritual development can progress very well with or without formal modes of worship. It can work either way.

The kind of bhakti we will explore in this book is the *up close and personal* kind. It is a non-sectarian approach that does not require any specific religious belief. For this kind of bhakti, you only need to become devoted to the possibilities within yourself.

Here, bhakti is about you, your nervous system, your desires, your practices, your spiritual experiences, and how it all plays out as you go out and engage in action in daily life. When we talk about bhakti as *love of God* here, what we mean is: What is our highest truth? What is the highest ideal we aspire to for ourselves? So far, maybe it is only a question we want to answer, like, "Is there more than this?"

If we ask the question in our heart with sincerity and give our emotions to it, we will have some good bhakti going. Real bhakti is very personal. It is about our innermost desire to become something more in our life. It is about wanting to know the truth, and using our emotions to move toward it. It can be a bare emotion – a deep hunger and wanting to know. It can express positively or negatively, and we can use either kind of emotion to propel our journey. This is bhakti.

Bhakti can also be very involved in a relationship with the icons and ideals of our religion. This is bhakti too, the kind we may have been exposed to and wondered about since childhood. For those who are inclined, there may be formal worship, prayer, invocation, chanting, ritual and other traditional devotional activities.

In whatever way it is occurring, the process of bhakti is the same – our emotions are willfully harnessed toward an ideal, which moves energy through our nervous system, purifying and opening it.

When longing is strongly expressed and then released in stillness deep within us, things happen. Answers start coming. *Practices* come to us. Then we begin to open and want to go higher. Then there will be more opening, more answers, more practices. Like that. Bhakti works like magic as it spirals up. It corresponds with the opening of our nervous system. The human nervous system is the gateway to the infinite.

We can see out into the infinite through our nervous system as it becomes purified. And God/Truth will manifest in our nervous system as increasing bhakti in our heart. God, the guru, and bhakti inside us are all the same thing. It is the infinite responding to our inner cry, coming in through the gateway of our nervous system.

Spiritual desire comes up naturally as our nervous system opens, and as our practices are married to our expanding desire. It is a personal process for each of us, yet it is quite easy to recognize in its different stages. Not abstract or nebulous at all.

Directed desire is the essential ingredient in all spiritual practices. It is bhakti that gets us to our meditation seat each day. Then we easily favor the procedure of our practice. Daily yoga practices are designed to open us up steadily over time. Then we have a constantly purifying and opening nervous system, a growing desire for truth and enlightenment, and we are always hankering to go to the next level of unfoldment. So it goes, up and up.

Ishta – The Chosen Ideal

While we know that desire leads to action, we also know that desire left on its own without the benefit of an underlying vision will be pulling us in many directions at the same time. Our emotion is a powerful fuel, but if it is not provided with a reliable channel for its expression through desire, not much good will come from it. The mind is also involved in this, because it is our emotions expressing as desires that inform the mind. From there, it is onward to action. So, you see, it all begins with how we point our emotions. It is about what we favor with our emotional energy. Desire is always seeking more, and it is up to us to provide that more in the form of an inspired vision.

In the first chapter, we used the word *vision* to represent the channel for desire leading to action. This implies that desire can be focused through a fixed lens. While in theory this is true, especially in worldly endeavors, it is a simplification when we consider the much broader scope of *human spiritual transformation*. In that case, we are not seeking a particular material outcome, but the purification and opening of the human nervous system so it can express its full potential.

In considering a systematic approach to bhakti, the cultivation of unending desire for spiritual realization, the concept of *ideal* provides the necessary flexibility. The Sanskrit word *Ishta* means *chosen ideal*, and offers the range of expression we need to travel the continuum of bhakti from where we are today to the highest reaches of devotion, and the resulting outpouring of divine love coming from within us.

What do we mean by *chosen ideal?* Our well-meaning religious institutions may interpret it to mean the god or ideal of our religion: Jesus, Krishna, Buddha, Allah, etc. This may be so if that is what resonates in our heart. But our chosen ideal can come in other forms also.

It can be a dedicated inquiry, such as, "Who am I, and what am I doing here?" Or the simple question, "Is there more than this that I am living now?"

It can be an affirmation, such as, "I will know the truth and the truth will set me free."

It can be an ideal of discrimination, such as, "This is truth, and this is not true."

And so on...

A chosen ideal is chosen by us, no one else. It is entirely personal. It can be a blend of ideals, such as the icons and ideals of our religion mixed with inquiry, affirmation and discrimination. And we will carry these through life, even as our ideal expands as we undergo the inner purification and opening associated with the ongoing process of human spiritual transformation.

Personality will play a role in one's chosen ideal. Those who are demonstratively devotional by nature may be inclined toward outer forms of devotion like worshipful conduct, singing, spiritual dancing, etc. Others who may be more analytical may be inclined toward introspection in stillness, self-inquiry and other less visible devotional acts.

Regardless of the choice of ishta, there will be devotion involved as we become committed to the course we have chosen. As our commitment deepens, our chosen ideal will evolve and change over time, according to our rising realization of truth. The more clearly we see what is emerging within us, the more concrete it will become, and our ideal will continue to evolve toward progressively more advanced stages.

Before the openings occur, there can be a tendency toward a more rigid view of the chosen ideal. This is certainly the case in most of the religions, where the ideal is often chosen for us rather than by us. And even in the individual there can be an inflexibility in the relationship with a chosen ideal. It is the difference between an icon representing a fixed view, or the same icon facilitating steadily expanding inner experience. Spiritual practices such as deep meditation and spinal breathing pranayama will unwind the rigidness that may be occurring in our relationship with a chosen ideal. Then a gradual shift in our relationship with our ideal can occur, according to need as inner awareness expands, with more inner silence moving in the outer expressions of our life.

As inner silence expands, our relationship with our ishta will expand also, through a constant gentle nudging coming from within. It is like the clothes we wear as we grow up. The bigger we become the bigger our clothes will become. Our ishta is like that too – infinitely expandable. The more we can see, the further our vision will reach beyond the limits we have known before. While we may have begun with a simple icon we derived from our religion, in the end, we may see our ishta encompassing the whole of humanity, and beyond to the entire universe. The larger our spirit becomes, the larger our ishta becomes, even if it is still represented by the same small icon on the altar of our devotion, whether it be a physical icon, or a non-physical ishta in our heart. It can be all of these.

Our ishta does not have to be fixed. In fact, it is good if we allow ourselves the flexibility to see our ideal as ever-expanding, even if still represented by a relatively fixed object or idea. The expansion is natural as we move along on our spiritual path. The expansion of our ishta is facilitated by a gentle favoring of our chosen ideal and the practices we will be inspired to undertake, rather than rigid concentration on ishta or means. We will find the greatest progress in favoring and releasing, favoring and releasing.

There is a paradox in this, and that is that the path of yoga is ultimately a path of release, of letting go. The doing we do in yoga is an undoing. When letting go into the divine flow becomes the ideal, the ideal itself will dissolve. That is when we have become the thing itself. This is the stage of abiding inner silence, ecstatic bliss, and outpouring divine love in unity. This is enlightenment. We arrive in this state through practices over the long term, so there is doing in this letting go.

Here are some general steps we may notice occurring as our chosen ideal evolves over time through the process of bhakti and yoga practices:

- Inspiration and questions – forming our ideal.
- Redirecting our energies of attraction and aversion.
- Adding practices for purification and opening.
- Expansion of stillness and the rise of ecstasy.
- Refining perception of divine experiences.
- Surrender to the transformation (kundalini).
- The inner process itself becoming the ideal.
- The ideal expanding outward to others.
- Service as the ideal – outpouring divine love.
- Unity – stillness in action in the field of *Oneness*.

These steps may tend to overlap and we may not experience each of them clearly. The evolution of our chosen ideal is a process resulting from our inner purification and opening, which will be unique to our nature, and dependent on our bhakti and the practices we undertake. Nevertheless, the stages of an evolving ishta will be more or less along the lines given above – beginning with our ideal forming around what inspires us, to increasingly more palpable experiences arising within and around us over time, which leave no doubt that great evolutionary forces are at work within us. As we expand from within, our ideal expands also, even as it becomes more real to us in every way.

So, an icon that inspires us, or a simple question like "Who am I?" asked with emotion, can lead to devotion to a high spiritual ideal, to many yoga practices, to a more peaceful and creative life, and ultimately to direct perception of the divine flow moving within and around us. It all leads to the divine seen as our own self in all who we may encounter. Then this becomes a life of personal self in sacred service to divine *Self*. It is an unending divine romance occurring within and all around us!

Our ishta evolves from a simple inspiration and longing for truth to the full expression of truth realized in daily living. The ideal continues to expand as we do. Throughout, we can have the same ishta we began with, in ever-expanding form, corresponding with our never-ending inner expansion. It is the journey of love and longing from separation to union. Through our evolution and the expansion of our view, we go beyond the bondage of orbiting opposites to the union of stillness in action. Then our ishta and our journey have become *One*.

The Systematic Transformation of Emotion

Once we have gotten a handle on our ishta, our chosen ideal, even just a glimmer of it, we will find ourselves in a position to bring the cosmic forces into alignment for manifesting that. If this seems like an exaggeration, it isn't.

The power of emotion is the power of the cosmos. Why? Because <u>all emotion is the power of love</u>, that which seeks to bind together all that exists. On this material plane, emotion may seem to be going in both directions – drawing us together in union, and pulling us apart in fear. But both of these are expressions of the same divine energy seeking fulfillment. It is only a misperception that repels us in fear, derision and the many other negatives that we see manifesting in the world. Emotion is always in search of love, either here or somewhere else if need be.

But we can transform the dynamic of emotion in the field of opposites to a much more productive purpose, and that is what our ishta gives us the ability to do. The power of the cosmos is brought into greatly increased resonance by devotion to our chosen ideal.

Much the way a martial artist can use the energy of his opponent to bring about the desired result, so too can emotional energy of all kinds be redirected to a higher purpose with the aid of our chosen ideal. Similarly, the many situations and relationships we encounter in our daily life can be used to transform our energies to a higher purpose, the purpose of our chosen ideal.

As we advance in our ability and habit to transform our emotions, great and small, to fulfill our chosen ideal, then we will find our devotion rising to a level of constant pouring. This pouring evolves over time to become automatic in all aspects of our life, with the end result being the constant outpouring of divine love.

This is what bhakti is, the constant pouring of desire toward our chosen ideal, which is ever-expanding the inner and outer dimensions of us. This is achieved by learning to transform all of our emotional energy for that. It does not mean ignoring our family and career. It means incorporating them, and everything in our life, into the process of transformation. In this way, our current activities and relationships rise to the level of divine interaction, and our devotion will soar with the consolidation of all emotional energy becoming divine desire.

As our ishta evolves, it will come to include our loved ones, which is very easy and natural because we are inclined this way with family and friends already. From there, our love will expand naturally to include others we encounter in our place of work, our community and the whole world.

The greater our devotion to others, the greater will the flow of divine energy through us become, further illuminating us and everyone around us.

Divine energy will be drawn to us no matter where we are. We will become a magnet to anyone who can aid in our inner flow, and they will be a magnet to us. By our own intention and acceptance, divine energy will flow. This is where the statement "Your faith has made you whole" comes from. It is the receiver of divine energy who determines the flow, not the source. Divine energy is everywhere, and can be easily found by one who is effectively transforming their emotional energy into pure bhakti. All the universe runs to support such a one.

Transforming Positive Emotional Energy

We all have positive emotional experiences occurring in our life. We have our loved ones, our friends, and the feelings gained from success we find in our endeavors in the world. All of these are opportunities for expanding our bhakti. Even the small feeling we gain from a tiny accomplishment (like emptying the trash) can be used to further our bhakti.

Before, we may have felt that feelings of love or accomplishment were a fulfillment in themselves, and we surely have sought to have more of them in our life. So we seek betterment in our relationships and in our work, so we can feel better more of the time.

But there is a hidden layer in all this, where there is much larger energy, a much larger fulfillment.

For example, consider the love of a child. To hold a small child, to have that feeling of nurturing and caring is beyond description for most of us. It is divine by definition. Yet, it can be taken even deeper than that with the use of our chosen ideal. If we do that, the child becomes an expression of our ishta and our holding of the child becomes divine worship. It may well have been anyway, for this is the nature of parenthood. It is natural for the parent-child relationship to be divine.

But will it seem so divine when the child becomes a "terrible two-year old," pulling the knick-knacks off the shelves and refusing to cooperate with the parent's requests? Or how about a full-blown adolescent in rebellion? Well, never mind the divine coddling then. But the love will not fade, even when it is expressing with firmness.

If we are on the path and have been cultivating our spiritual desire, our relationship will continue to be divine, expressing as needed through all the ups and downs of life, rooted in inner silence. This will have a profound effect on our own development, as well as on our children, who will instinctively know that something is operating beyond the diversions of the moment. Something positive, something that will outlast every mishap that may be encountered in life. It is a knowing that our children will carry with them all through life. Divine love is very practical in this way. Once it has touched us, it will never leave us.

While we can take every positive emotion and elevate it to divine status by incorporating it into our chosen ideal, so too can we do the same with emotions associated with the so-called negative experiences we encounter in life. The truth is, there is no such thing as a negative experience. It is only by our coloring of perceptions that positive and negative exist. It is we who identify what is positive and negative. We always have a choice. As we advance on the path of bhakti and with the powerful spiritual practices it will inspire, we will know that there is a reality beyond all the positives and negatives of life. It is a reality of abiding inner silence, ecstatic bliss, and outpouring divine love.

Both positive and negative emotions can be taken to the extreme in terms of bhakti, to the point of emotional frenzy, and beyond. This is a characteristic which has been documented in the lives of the saints and sages. The great ones have used both positive and negative emotions, every feeling they had, applied to the divine quest. Is such emotional desperation necessary to travel the path to enlightenment? It depends on the person.

Famous sages like Rumi, Ramakrishna, Buddha and Jesus had this in common. The more inspired and/or desperate they became, the more they expressed the divine within them. At times they may have been regarded to be mad for God or Truth. If we are to be mad for something let it be for that. Divine experience is a mixture of ecstatic joy, fear and tears, all for the singular unswerving purpose of fulfilling our chosen ideal.

Transforming Negative Emotional Energy

It may not always be obvious that we have a choice in how our emotions are directed and focused. So often we are caught up in the events of the moment and our emotional energy becomes focused in nonproductive ways due to knee-jerk reactions. But these can be changed through the methods of bhakti.

For example, let's suppose we are stuck in a traffic jam, and are late for an appointment. The longer we are stuck, the more our emotions may tend to rise about our increasing lateness. The knee-jerk reaction in this case may be to lean on the horn and curse out the window at someone who has cut us off to gain a car-length or two in the huge mass of traffic creeping along the highway slower than a walk. On the other hand, if we have a chosen ideal for our spiritual evolution that is becoming strong in us, we will be able to take the emotional energy rising in us due to the traffic and lateness and transform it to cry for our spiritual evolution. Instead of honking and yelling at the driver who has cut us off, we complain to the divine about our slow progress toward enlightenment.

"Oh Lord, my journey to realization of Thee is going so slowly!"

Yes, complaining with heart-felt emotion to God (however we may conceive Him/Her/It) can be very productive, as long as we are willing to act to resolve what it is we are complaining about. Our frustration about being stuck and late in traffic can be easily redirected to be frustration for being stuck and late on our spiritual path. What is the benefit in this?

While honking our horn and yelling out the car window will do little to speed up the traffic jam, expressing intense emotion toward our chosen spiritual ideal can have a dramatic effect on our spiritual progress. The effects can be both tangible and intangible, as long as we are open to what may come. Bhakti is not about unloading our perceived troubles. It is about opening the divine doorway within us.

In the tangible sense, as we are lamenting our lateness in the traffic jam, that is, our spiritual lateness, the redirected emotional energy may go toward us resolving to put in extra effort to seek knowledge of spiritual practices that we may have been putting off for some time. Or to become more regular in our daily meditation and other sitting practices and not miss them as often as we did before.

In the intangible sense, we may have a revelation of new spiritual knowledge right then and there in the traffic jam. It can happen. Or we may encounter the knowledge we need to take next the steps on our path in a mysterious way – maybe we pull off the highway in frustration, go into a café, and meet someone who provides exactly what we need to take the next step on our path. It happens often to people who are steadily building devotion in relation to their chosen ideal. More bhakti brings many small miracles into our life – and some big ones too.

This is not to promote a superstitious approach to spiritual development. It is not to encourage the seeking of "signs" in everything that happens in our life. We don't have to be trying to "read the tea leaves" to find our salvation. If we attend to the necessary causes, the effects will be there.

If we are favoring the redirection of our emotional energy and the transformation of our everyday desires toward our chosen ideal, then what we need for our spiritual fulfillment will find us in one way or another. If we take care of devotion and are willing to act when the appropriate opportunities present themselves, then the knowledge and tools we need will find us.

Much of what we have been saying before now may seem to assume that everyone will be enthusiastic about their spiritual prospects, have a clear chosen ideal and be moving along converting all their emotional energy at a good pace. Of course this is not going to be the case for everyone all the time. But we do know that everyone has an emotional life, even if that is being expressed as an inclination to not be enthusiastic or excited about anything. Those who are conspicuously disinterested or running away from life will have their emotional energy invested in that disinterest and running away, and that energy can be transformed to serve an ideal, whatever that ideal may be. The ideal does not have to be flashy, or even obvious. It may be as modest as making the time to meditate twice daily, which is not a small thing at all. It surely will lead to openings, and the bhakti will expand along with it. The main thing is to understand that every feeling we have can be applied in a direction that we choose. The energy we may be expending to run away in fear or guilt is of equal value in bhakti as the energy we may be expending for seeking. Whether our negative or positive emotions are invisible or very intense and expressed outwardly, we can use them all for a chosen higher purpose – our enlightenment.

Bhakti with Balance – Self-Pacing

It was mentioned earlier that the power of the cosmos becomes focused in one who is engaged in the systematic cultivation of bhakti. Whether this is true in the absolute sense may be subject to debate. However, there can be no doubt that tremendous forces are released in us as we travel the path of spiritual purification and opening. This will be seen occurring within our nervous system and neurobiology, and around us in our physical environment. It is the process of *human spiritual transformation.*

The press for progress will become especially strong when our bhakti leads us to undertake powerful spiritual practices such as deep meditation, spinal breathing pranayama and additional methods that are covered in detail in the AYP writings. But even with bhakti alone, we may find ourselves overwhelmed with the openings that present themselves. Sometimes we may get more than we have bargained for, and it is important to understand that we always have a choice in what we undertake, and in what we can let go by. Bhakti and other yoga practices bring change in powerful inward ways, and we will be wise to navigate the causes and effects in our practice to maintain good progress with comfort and safety. This is called *self-pacing* in practice.

How do we self-pace our bhakti? It is simple really. All we must do is put our attention on other things. Doing this can also be regarded as *grounding*, in that we bring our energies back to earth by focusing on more mundane things rather then the elevating influence of our chosen ideal. So instead of stirring our divine longing into a fever pitch to the point where it becomes destabilizing for us, we can go for a long walk or do some grounding activity like working in the garden.

Another way to self-pace our bhakti is to serve others in ordinary ways – like helping a friend in need with simple things like running errands, cleaning up if they are not able, or whatever. Nothing fancy or blazing with devotion. Just the ordinary things.

We can always go back to our blazing bhakti at any time we choose. We just want to avoid getting too carried away, to the point of losing touch with everyday activities, and possibly compromising our health. This can slow our progress by exhausting our neurobiology, and hamper our ability to engage in daily spiritual practices. When the experiences become too intense, it is wise to regard it all as *scenery*, and just carry on with the ordinary things. The energy released within us due to bhakti can become extremely powerful, and even more so with a full battery of daily spiritual practices being utilized.

Think of bhakti combined with powerful spiritual practices as being like a fast sports car on a long and sometimes winding road. On the straight-aways we will be inclined to push down on the accelerator to speed up. But what will we do when the road begins to wind around sharp curves on a mountain? If we keep our foot pressed down on the accelerator then, we could end up flying off a cliff. Bhakti and yoga practices are a lot like this. When purification and opening are going smoothly, we can move along at a good pace with comfort and safety. But when purification and opening are reaching a level that challenges our neurobiology, then this is the time to ease up on the accelerator, self-pace our practices, beginning with our desire to be doing more and more in yoga. It will usually be best to gently favor our tendency toward bhakti at a nice safe pace, rather than be going whole-hog for an overdose of inner purification and opening, which can set us back for weeks or months as we recover from the excess.

Times have changed. No longer are we spiritual paupers, scraping for every little bit of knowledge, method of practice, and inner purification and opening we can find. A little bhakti goes a long way in these times of rapid openings. A great wealth of knowledge and practices will be coming to us with just a little longing. More than we can handle if we try and say "yes" to all of it. We have been hungry for so long, and maybe we will eat too much at first. Then we will be learning how to self-pace for best results.

One of the key lessons we will learn is how to balance our bhakti with our common sense. The vast force of the cosmic evolution will not always have our physical comfort and health in mind as it seeks our transformation. It will want it all right now, and that is not possible. It takes time for the nervous system to undergo the necessary inner purification and opening, so we must pace ourselves, or face difficulties and delays in our progress. If a long-distance runner goes too fast and strains a muscle, she will have to stop long enough to heal before she can resume the race. If she paces herself, she will finish the race much sooner. It is like that on the spiritual path also.

There is also the matter of meeting our responsibilities in life. Our ever-increasing bhakti, will open many possibilities to us. Some of these will be practical within the lifestyle we have been living, including being compatible with responsibilities we may have to family and community. Other possibilities may not be compatible with our present lifestyle, calling for a radical change at great cost to those who depend on us. If we are the family breadwinner and are suddenly inclined to leave everyone and permanently go off to the mountaintop, we will be wise to let that impulse go. Maybe do a few spiritual retreats on holidays instead, and not desert the family for our own salvation. There was a time when this sort of conduct was considered noble. This is no longer true. There are more than enough resources available now for everyone to travel the spiritual path in rapid fashion without leaving responsibilities behind.

In fact, having responsibilities in ordinary life provides a great advantage to those with increasing bhakti, because there are many opportunities to expand the chosen ideal into a much broader field of action. Sitting practices can be added into the daily routine, and this will accelerate our bhakti dramatically. Then all of our activities and relationships will rise to become modes of service, which is the natural evolution of *karma yoga*, leading to freedom and fulfillment in everyday life. Responsibilities are not in opposition to our spiritual development. If we travel our spiritual path while living an ordinary life, fulfilling our responsibilities will become the fruition of our spiritual unfoldment, and our subsequent influence for positive change in the world will become much greater.

So, it will be wise to balance our bhakti with good common sense. With the powerful spiritual practices we have available for everyone nowadays, we no longer have to be desperate for running away with every opening that may present itself. It will happen a few times, and we will learn. We will have more openings than we can pursue with good progress and safety. We can choose the blend of bhakti and practices that is most compatible with our inclinations and the life we are living. This is *self-directed spiritual practice*. There will be more than enough positive change occurring within the life we are already living. Enlightenment is happening here and now, and we can do it. It is not more likely to be occurring somewhere else in some other way. It is here!

Ponder that, and transform your feelings about it to enliven your chosen ideal. There are many things we can do to enhance our spiritual progress. We will look at some of those now.

Bhakti and the Limbs of Yoga

Centuries ago, a short scripture was written by the Indian sage, *Patanjali*, systematizing a range of practices for stimulating the natural capabilities inherent within every human nervous system for purification and opening, leading to realization of the condition we call *enlightenment*.

Patanjali's scripture is called the *Yoga Sutras* (meaning, "stitches of union"), and it provides one of the world's clearest summaries of the methods and experiences of human spiritual transformation.

The integrated practices offered by Patanjali comprise the famous *Eight Limbs of Yoga*. This list is so complete in its coverage of human spiritual capabilities that is can serve as a check-list for assessing the completeness of literally any spiritual path.

Patanjali's Eight Limbs of Yoga include:

- **Yama** (*restraints* – non-violence, truthfulness, non-stealing, preservation and cultivation of sexual energy, and non-covetousness)
- **Niyama** (*observances* – purity, contentment, spiritual intensity, study of spiritual knowledge and *Self*, and active surrender to the divine)
- **Asana** (postures and physical maneuvers)
- **Pranayama** (breathing techniques)
- **Pratyahara** (introversion of the senses)
- **Dharana** (systematic attention on an object)
- **Dhyana** (meditation – systematic dissolving of the object in consciousness)
- **Samadhi** (absorption in pure bliss consciousness)

There is an additional category of practice called **Samyama**, which utilizes the last three limbs of yoga in a systematic manner to stimulate an endless outpouring of divine love in daily life, which is the rise of *stillness in action* – the ongoing ecstatic union of inner and outer life. Happiness!

The role of bhakti in the limbs of yoga is pervasive. In finding the inspiration to consider an integration of methods as comprehensive as the eight limbs of yoga, we will first have bhakti, a desire to fulfill our highest potential. Then we will work our way through building a daily routine of practices, step-by-step, moved by our bhakti (the limbs of yoga are not necessarily taken in the order listed). And, in the end, we will fly on the wings of bhakti as we share our love and ever-expanding spiritual influence with all, near and far, who we see as expressions of our divine *Self*.

Throughout this process, our bhakti will be expanding due to the onward march of purification and opening within us. The growth of our spiritual desire is none other than the growth of stillness within us and the divine flow coming through us. Bhakti and the emerging spiritual reality are one and the same. It is the divine flow of life that is always seeking the union of the absolute stillness of pure bliss consciousness with the energetic expressions of life within and around us. These two (stillness and energetic ecstasy), fully integrated and lived in *Oneness*, constitute the wholeness of life in the enlightened condition.

Bhakti shows up clearly in the language of the eight limbs of yoga in *Niyama*, the observances, as spiritual intensity (*tapas*) and active surrender to the divine (*ishvara pranidhana*).

The intensity of our surrender to our chosen ideal, our *hunger and thirst* for the divine, is an essential dynamic of bhakti leading to all spiritual progress, including undertaking daily practices such as deep meditation, spinal breathing pranayama, physical methods such as asanas, mudras and bandhas, the preservation and cultivation of sexual energy (tantra), and an ongoing inquiry into the nature of our *Self*.

With engagement in daily practices such as those mentioned, and ultimately all of the limbs on the tree of yoga, purification and opening will be greatly accelerated, and our bhakti will be expanded as part of this overall process.

All of the limbs of yoga are naturally interconnected within the human nervous system. Each practice we undertake influences the effectiveness of all other practices. This is true of bhakti as well. Bhakti increases the effectiveness of deep meditation and spinal breathing pranayama, and these practices increase the effectiveness of bhakti. If we cultivate our bhakti and are meditating daily, we naturally become more inclined toward spiritual study, and so on. It is like that with the interconnectedness of all yoga practices. The whole of yoga is much greater than the sum of its parts, just as the whole human nervous system is much greater than its individual parts. Yoga and the spiritual capabilities of the human being are one and the same. Yoga is derived directly from the higher functioning our nervous system, not invented somehow apart from it.

Bhakti in the overall functioning of yoga fuels the expanding spiral of desire, action in practices, purification and opening, more desire, more action in practices, more purification and opening, and so on...

Where does it all lead? To a permanent state of abiding inner silence, ecstatic bliss, outpouring divine love, and the unification of limited personal self with unlimited divine *Self*. And then bhakti goes on as we continue to express in the world in ways that are unifying for all who we encounter.

An essential aspect of bhakti is found in our willingness to act upon our surging divine desire in practical ways. Engaging in daily sitting practices is the epitome of this, because effective practices, undertaken consistently over the long term, will do more than any other kind of action to accelerate our bhakti and our overall progress toward enlightenment. Engaging in practices in combination with our bhakti is so effective that we will find ourselves in the luxurious position of having to slow down at times. It is possible to have too much of a good thing. So we self-pace our practices and bhakti as necessary, as discussed previously. Self-pacing is an aspect of practices that is discussed throughout the AYP writings.

At times, the question may arise, "I don't feel intense spiritual desire, and am doing yoga practices anyway. So where is my bhakti?"

If we have found the commitment to do our daily yoga practices, forming and sustaining the habit, then bhakti is there. It may not always be in the form of intense hunger and thirst for the divine, or gushing spiritual emotions. In fact, a quiet resolve on our path is equal or greater bhakti than the kind that is demonstrating itself dramatically all the time. At the heart of our spiritual development is the rise of inner silence. This is cultivated in daily deep meditation, but can also be resident in us to a degree prior to consciously stepping onto our spiritual path. Stillness is bhakti and bhakti is stillness.

Bhakti is also energy, just as stillness underlies and animates all energy. Emotion is the movement of energy within us, moving to fulfill desires deep in our heart. In time, the energetic side of bhakti is experienced as whole body *ecstatic conductivity* and radiance, which is the awakening of *kundalini*, the vast latent evolutionary energy residing within us. This gives rise to the introversion of sensory perception (pratyahara, the fifth limb of yoga), and a more intimate relationship with the divine flowing within and around us. The experience of ecstasy rising is very noticeable, and sometimes overwhelming, consuming us in a vast inner column of fiery luminous energy, inevitably radiating outward from us. Our bhakti plays a key role in the advancement of inner energy flow, and is also influenced by the events occurring inside us. Our ishta expands accordingly, always reaching beyond current experiences, no matter how dramatic they may be. A true ishta will never rest on its laurels for long. It always seeks the highest in us.

So, the range of experiences we can have with bhakti is diverse and profound – from the dispassion of abiding inner silence (the *witness*) to the intense emotions of direct perception of the divine flow occurring everywhere. All of this is based in our desire for opening, and the means we are inspired to employ to promote the process of human spiritual transformation within us.

All action in practices that we undertake as a result of our bhakti is in the field of *karma yoga*, the realm of causes and effects. Practices, and how we integrate them, constitute an optimization of causes and effects for the purpose of our spiritual unfoldment. Because this is building a relationship of actions and reactions within us that is predictable and repeatable by anyone on their own path, we can say that it is a scientific approach to human spiritual transformation.

Karma yoga also looks beyond our structured spiritual practices to our conduct in every aspect of daily life. This is the most common way karma yoga is viewed. But when viewed as beginning with sitting practices, karma yoga takes on a new dimension. Just as rising spiritual desire is a good launching platform for entry into practices, so too are practices a good launching platform for elevating our conduct in daily living. In short, the longing for fulfillment in our heart (our bhakti) is a direct route to the meditation seat, and the meditation seat is a direct route to increasingly evolutionary action in the world. This is an effective approach for undertaking karma yoga, which we will delve into next.

Chapter 3 – Karma Yoga

The word *Karma* has become a cliché in our society, sometimes put in humorous terms relating to the foibles and mishaps that occur in everyday life:

"I tripped and fell down. It must be my karma."

"I did that foolish thing, and I'll do it again. It's not my fault. It's my karma."

On the serious side, the concept of karma may be affixed to tragedies as heart-rending as the loss of a loved one, or a natural disaster that takes hundreds or thousands of lives. How can one word explain such inexplicable events? It can't really. Yet, there is something in the word *karma* that rings deep in the psyche of all of us. It has to do with our sense of destiny, fate, or what seems beyond our knowing. When we can find no other reason, we may seek a hidden logic.

But, while karma may have something to do with destiny and fate, it is also beyond beliefs we may harbor that cross over into the realm of superstition. If karma is superstition, it is only because people have needed to see it in that light in attempts to explain the unexplainable.

On the other hand, karma is the working principle of *cause and effect* operating in life that can be of great practical utility on our spiritual path, if we view it in that context. When we do, karma can be elevated to the level of practice. When that occurs, we call it *Karma Yoga*, which means *divine union through action*.

Karma means *action and its consequences*.

"As you sow, so shall you reap."

Yet, so often, we use the term with resignation, only in relation to the consequences: "This thing that is happening is our karma," etc.

However, <u>karma is both cause and effect</u>, so it stands to reason that the effects can be altered in some way by influencing underlying causes. There is something we can do about the consequences aspect of our karma, and, for that matter, about the karma of the world. Therefore, nothing is necessarily predestined or a product of fate. We can act to bring about more positive consequences for ourselves, and for everyone. This is the promise of karma yoga.

How can we do that? The power lies in each of us, and in the choices we make.

Action and its Consequences

We are all familiar with the basic mechanics of desire, action and the resulting consequences.

If we want to become a doctor, we go to school for a long time, and, in the end, we become a doctor. Desire, action, consequences.

What we may not have considered in the beginning is the multitude of ramifications associated with the path we have chosen. It is not possible to know everything beforehand. But we do the best we can in following a course that we feel is in line with our desire. If it is our unwavering passion to become a doctor, then, whatever obstacles we may encounter on our journey, we will find ways to overcome them. Such is the power of having a clear vision, a chosen ideal. If there is such a thing as destiny, our vision and persistence will define it. Destiny is in our deepest longing.

In this kind of scenario, the workings of karma seem pretty clear. We choose a course and work steadily toward our goal.

But are the workings of karma really so clear?

The Unfathomable Consequences of Karma

If we throw a stone in a pond, can we know the full effects it will have? Can we trace the effect of every ripple going out, and the effect of every ripple coming back from the opposite bank? Perhaps we can if we develop a mathematical model that is sufficiently sophisticated.

It has been said that the flapping of a butterfly's wings will influence the most distant star. Can we predict the results of that?

Astrologers spend their careers doing something like that, attempting to determine the influence of the gravitational forces of the planets and stars in our lives. Is it possible? The best astrologers might be right a little more than half the time, so there is something to it. But is this enough to say that we can know the consequences of karma in the cosmic sense?

Likewise, it is said that the influences in our lives that may defy logical explanation are the result of actions we have undertaken in *past lives*, the result of our numerous incarnations in bodily form – our karmic tendencies sown in a distant past we no longer remember. Is this a good argument for reincarnation?

It does offer a rationale for the inexplicable events we may experience in life, and the apparent gifts and handicaps that innocent children may arrive with at birth. But can we really know for sure? Should we be spending our precious time looking back into the murky realms of past lives to understand reasons for what is happening in our lives today? If we work at it long enough, we may find some clarity. But, for the most part, it will be unfathomable, like gazing at star charts, or pondering the effects of stones thrown in ponds, or the whisperings of butterfly wings traveling across the universe.

Our destiny may be hidden in the stars, but the rest will be up to us through the choices we make each day to forward our spiritual progress. We can watch for the lingering effects of ancient events, taking the role of spectator, or we can act in ways that directly influence all outcomes in the here and now, taking the role of participant.

The Myth of Sin

What is sin? If you look it up in the dictionary, you will see it focuses on the negative aspects of "As you sow, so shall you reap," or karma.

Sin is defined as, "An offense against religious or moral law, an offense against God."

Sowing and reaping is one thing, a process of nature. It just happens as we act in ways that are either in the direction of or away from purifying our nervous system and expressing divine love. What we put in is what we get out. If we do yoga practices and favor opening over closing, we give ourselves a big advantage in this process.

Sin is a step outside the natural process of "as you sow..." and karma. It is an *offense*. An offense to who? Sin is colored with human judgement. If you do thus-and-so, you commit sin. You are doing bad. You are offending God. Who decides this? Most often, it is we who decide it through our guilt and shame over our actions. Maybe we have been conditioned by others since childhood to feel that way about ourselves. In our still-limited state of awareness we tend to act in ways that bind us, and in our conscience (the divine morality in us) we feel remorse. If we do not judge ourselves, others will certainly be there to do it for us. In doing so, they place themselves in the position of intermediary between us and our salvation. And there you have it, the psychological structure that holds most of the world's organized religions together.

The concept of sin is a human coloring of natural law. Sin is a spin on a process of nature. It rises out of our guilt and/or someone else's judgment. Sin is a myth.

Overindulgence in the concept of sin can lead to a sense of hopelessness, and an unhealthy dependence on others for our salvation, when, in truth, there is only one place we will ever find it, within ourselves.

Expecting someone else, ordained or not, to relieve us of our sins is a formula for failure. Spiritual life is not a business transaction where we give this and get that. It does not happen like that.

Surrendering to our chosen high ideal, our ishta, is something else. It is a private matter in our heart, not subject to anyone else's scrutiny or judgement. As long as we are letting go for a higher ideal deep in our heart, our bhakti will have great purifying power, and draw us to spiritual practices.

If we have been trained to see ourselves as hopeless sinners, it will be wise to reconsider it carefully. For if we do not believe in our own divinity, it will be difficult to find the desire necessary to make the journey home. Our identity as sinners is a label we put on ourselves, while our identity as divine beings is a demonstrable human condition we can claim as our own.

Saints and saviors over thousands of years have demonstrated again and again the ability we all have for human spiritual transformation.

Sitting to meditate for the first time can shatter the illusory grip of sin. It won't free us completely from all inner obstructions on the first day, but it is the beginning of a road we can travel that will reveal increasing divine light as we purify and open our nervous system further each day.

Transcending Karma and Putting It to Good Use

While, on the one hand, it is not possible to fathom the full consequences of karma, on the other hand it is quite possible to influence all outcomes of karma through our actions. We have a choice about how we view the world and what we do in our life each day. The actions we choose to undertake will have short term and long term consequences.

Our choices will be colored by the many influences in our lives (unfathomable karma!), and the ingrained habits we live by, so we might question whether our supposed *free will* is an illusion. Do we really have a choice about the things we do? If we have given the time and effort to strengthen a higher ideal in our life, we will have a choice. Our ideal, our ishta, will be our choice. From that, everything else will flow. This is the vital connection between bhakti and the actions we undertake, which determine our relationship to the karmic machinery of cause and effect that is constantly operating in life.

Whether our chosen ideal is for God or for Truth, in whatever form we may be drawn to, the effect will be the same. Ideals like these reach beyond the limiting aspects of karma. Having a high ideal is the sure way to reach beyond whatever limitations we are facing in life. Devotion to a high ideal is the way by which we can transcend karma, even while we are making good use of its underlying principles.

There is free will. However, exercising it effectively requires some finesse. If our chosen ideal inspires us to make choices that take us beyond the influences that distract us, then we will be on our way.

Developing bhakti in relation to our chosen ideal is the first step. Then we will be presented with opportunities and act in ways that promote the process of our spiritual development. In the AYP approach, we use an integrated system of practices, beginning with deep meditation. This first step in practice is a key one, once we have found the will to act on our spiritual desire.

With deep meditation, we are cultivating the natural presence of inner silence within ourselves, an abiding stillness that penetrates all of our thoughts, feelings and actions. This innate stillness, also referred to as *pure bliss consciousness*, is beyond the ups and downs of life. Life goes on as it did before, but stillness resides in us as a *silent witness* that we recognize as our own self. As we come to know our *Self* beyond the many influences in our life, it has a profound effect on the way we view events. We see life occurring as change on the ocean of our stillness. Even catastrophic events will be unable to touch us in our deepest realm of *Self-awareness*.

This is the transcendence of karma. It is not the elimination of karma. Karma will go on, but our relationship with it will change, and it's role in our life will change also.

Once we have begun daily deep meditation, we will be on the road to becoming the master of karma, rather than its servant. When we act from the perspective of inner silence, our actions will be capable of transforming the influences of karma in ways that are evolutionary and joyfully liberating, rather than in ways that are darkly limiting. For one who is awakening in the fullness of expanding inner silence, the mechanics of karma become a vehicle for spiritual development. Likewise, the expansion of inner silence through daily deep meditation, provides for constant expansion of bhakti. It is a cycle of desire, action and consequences leading to a life of ever-expanding peace, creativity, and joyous service.

This shift is a gradual one, occurring over years of daily deep meditation, increasing bhakti and the normal course of our life's activities. Steadily, our actions in daily life rise to the level of divine relationship. While, before, we may have spent significant energy attempting to either reclaim or change the past, we now spend our time in the present, enjoying what is, and engaging in conduct that is both immediately fulfilling and sowing the seeds for a better future. Both our past and future can be made better by living increasingly in the now.

We do not do this by trying to. It cannot be done that way. We can't will an immediate shift in our quality of life, because the life we are living has been structured in us for a long time. But we can gradually unwind the structures within us through the power of bhakti and yoga practices. And, in doing so, we can transform our relationship with karma. Karma will not be eliminated. It will be transformed. There is the idea that karma can be erased, made to go away. This is not so. As long as we have action, we will have consequences, the process of karma. But we can transform karma's influence to be uplifting and divine – this is just as true for so-called negative karma as it is for so-called positive karma. The fact that consequences are coming to us from past actions does not mean any particular coloring comes with it. It is we in the present who do the coloring. All karma can be seen as being for good or ill. As our inner silence grows and matures, all karma will become a positive springboard to new openings in spirit.

This is not a passive experience. It is not the killing off of desires. It is the transformation of desire to divine purpose. Then we find that our ever-seeking desire has been the *guru* in us all along, carrying us steadily forward into fullness. Then all events become opportunities.

The blend of bhakti, spiritual practices like deep meditation, and our actions in ordinary life, leads to a harmonizing of influences sown in the past, and the fulfillment of openings in the future. It is all happening in the now. While it has been said that we should be "Be here now," this can be expanded to say, "Be and do here now."

Our active devotion to our chosen ideal is what makes the difference. Once we have realized our abiding inner silence, we can make good use of karma, no matter what it is bringing us in life.

The Spiritual Evolution of Action

We are conditioned in our consumer culture to believe that if we want something, we can just go to the store and buy it. At the same time we know that anything worth having is worth working for. Going to the store to buy something we want may be the culmination of a long time of saving enough money to do that. Of course, many things are bought on credit these days, so there is the illusion of instant gratification.

Fortunately, we can't buy enlightenment on credit. We have to earn it through our bhakti and persistent dedication to daily practice. Then we will have something that transcends the limitations of time and space. We become *That*.

While spiritual maturity is only about living in the now, it takes time to arrive at where we already are. There can be many instances of instant gratification along the way, if not the whole thing. Life with spiritual practices in the picture will be improving step-by-step, with many small miracles occurring – and some big ones too.

So it will be with our actions in daily living. While we'd like to see our actions instantly elevated to the level of enlightenment, it is a journey – an evolution. As with all evolution, we begin where we are today, and take the next step. And, ultimately, the gaining of enlightenment is giving it away. The less we need it, the more of it we will have. Until then, our journey will be an evolutionary cycle of desire, action and opening, leading to more desire, action and opening.

Going in Circles and Traveling in a Straight Line

Before spiritual practices, our journey will tend to be circular, at least from the standpoint of spiritual progress. We may lead a very productive life in the material sense, build up a big bank account, have many material things, and so on. But, at the end, we will feel like we did in the beginning – wanting something more.

There is always time for spiritual progress, even with our last breath. But because human spiritual transformation is a journey of inner purification and opening, it behooves us to start as early as possible and make the best use of the time we have. Rome was not built in a day!

The first truly evolutionary step in our action is to undertake daily practices. It is not such a big thing – only a few minutes of sitting in deep meditation morning and evening. That is all it takes to get the ball rolling. Of course, before we make the commitment to practices, there must be the desire, some bhakti stirring inside – something within us that says, "There must be more than this."

If we act on it, we will find out that there is more – a lot more.

So the evolution of action begins in earnest with a commitment to daily spiritual practices. Then we will find ourselves moving in a forward direction as inner silence begins to rise within us. Then it is a new ball game. We go from traveling in circles to traveling more in a straight line in the direction our inner longing takes us. The straight line is a cycle also, an ever-widening one of purification and opening.

Eventually we will transcend the longing itself, and divine energy will be flowing outward from us instead of the wanting flowing constantly inward. That is when we will have crossed the tipping point of enlightenment, when the inner flow has shifted and we are no longer seeking it, but giving it away!

Then the cycle of desire and action takes on a new dynamic – a constant outpouring of the divine. The outpouring is its own journey, and its own destination. The label *enlightenment* may be stamped on it by outside observers, but there will be no proclamation from the one who is fully engaged in it.

There is no one to proclaim, except the flow of *Love* itself.

Mapping the Spiritual Evolution of Action

So, how does it happen, this so-called evolution of action? Can we map it out so there can be some idea of what to expect?

Well, everyone is different in how purification and opening occurs in the nervous system. But there is a general progression we may notice as we move along. It is first related to our mind, and how we perceive our own thoughts, feelings and the world around us. As experiences advance, there an opening up of these perceptions that will determine our actions in the world. The process of transformation has to do with the rise of inner silence and how we see things as our sense of self moves beyond the objects of our perception to naturally reside in our abiding inner silence, or the *witness*.

Our actions play upon this expanding inner silence and are affected accordingly. Consider these stages of mind that evolve as we engage in daily spiritual practices over time, and how our actions will be influenced as we progress through each stage:

- Pre-Witnessing – Action based on external desires for satisfying the body-based personal self.

- Witnessing – Action perceived as separate from our emerging silent self. A sense of doing without doing.

- Discrimination – A creative morality radiating from stillness which we can choose to manifest in our actions. A heightened sense of conscience.

- Passionate Dispassion – Moving beyond conscious discrimination to the automatic expression of inner values in our actions.

- Outpouring Divine Love – Joyful service without the need to receive in return. Ongoing realization of truth in ordinary life. Divine romance and the unfoldment of unity.

As mentioned, everyone will find the experience on their journey to be a little different. But there are certain elements we all have in common. Without these, progress will be limited. The constants involved in this process are daily practices (deep meditation especially), rising inner silence (the *witness*), and a gradual shift from intention and action based in outer events, outcomes and time scales, to intention and action based internally in stillness (samyama), which naturally leads to more harmonious outcomes always occurring in the present. Our desires are elevated accordingly as the opening progresses, being part of the shift from limited self-awareness to the emerging broader awareness of unity. As this occurs, stillness becomes dynamic in our awareness, culminating in the constant outpouring of divine love and the realization of unity in all action. This is the fruition of human spiritual transformation.

The result is, "Do unto others as we would have them do unto us."

The unity experience is ourselves doing for others who are perceived to also be ourselves. We find ourselves to be mirrored in the many flavors of life everywhere we go, and great love and joy is found in helping. It is life in *Oneness*.

Then every action becomes an offering, an act of devotion (bhakti). There is no pomp about it. The ceremony is found in the simple act of living our life as we did before, and sharing along the way. It is life lived in peace, with progress at every step. Then the machinery of karma is always operating for the greater good, with every action and every consequence being a stepping-stone to new openings.

There will be overlap in the stages of mind we experience along our path. For example, in pre-witnessing stage, we will not be entirely without a sense of the witness, or without a conscience to aid us in making moral choices, to greater or lesser degree. Some of our choices will be automatic – we will do the right thing without fanfare, and our love will flow to the dear ones in our life, bringing us a sense of unity. Everyone has these experiences, and all the stages of mind are included: pre-witnessing, witnessing, discrimination, passionate dispassion, and outpouring divine love.

Even someone who has never sat to meditate will have these overlaps. The elements of enlightened living are present in all of us right now. We only need to reveal the capabilities we already have.

As we become inspired to tap our greater potential, as we become devoted to a higher ideal of our choosing, and act day after day on that, then all of these stages will become increasingly illuminated over time. The order given will still be there, because each stage relies on the previous stage for full development.

Before we can discriminate between inner-based and outer-based action we will need an inner relationship in stillness from which to be choosing from – *the witness*. Until we have a sense of an abiding inner witness (cultivated in deep meditation), we cannot choose to reside in it as we engage in action. We can't create the witness by a mental act. We can only have the witness through meditation. In the language of yoga, the witness is *samadhi*, and it is stabilized through the process of meditation. The witness is a condition of our inner neurobiology which is cultivated over time, not an attitude or idea we can conjure up at will if it has not been cultivated over time through daily deep meditation.

Likewise, we cannot have the full flowering of passionate dispassion until we have developed the habit of discrimination – making choices based in stillness. As we progress in developing the habit of discrimination, then the process of discrimination itself will gradually dissolve into stillness, becoming dispassion. As we continue, carried forward by our bhakti, we will find that we can be passionate and dispassionate at the same time as we continue to act in ordinary daily life. Dispassion is not a static condition. Even as we reside in stillness, we can move with great passion. This is the paradox of rising enlightenment.

There is no place to stop and say, "Now it is done, and there is nothing more to do."

Spirit is forever in motion, forever creating and forever serving. *We are That – Stillness in Action.* We cannot be an incarnation of *Love* and cease acting for the benefit of the whole of existence.

The surest way to transcend karma and get off the wheel of birth and death is by consciously becoming an expression of life's purpose, which is the realization of the divine nature of life in all actions, great and small. The undoing of bondage on the material plane is found in doing without doing.

Karma yoga is fulfilled when we have become stillness in action. Then we can do without doing, laugh without laughing, and cry without crying. We will be everything, even while we are nothing.

Then we are free, and in the best position to serve, with all of our actions naturally aligned with the force of cosmic evolution.

The Role of Service

It has been said that the path of service is a royal road to enlightenment. And even if it isn't, it does much good in the world, so favoring helping others will always be a worthy endeavor.

But is service alone really a path to enlightenment? What is its role in fulfilling our ultimate spiritual aspirations?

There have been some famous people who spent a lifetime in service to others, engaged in *right action*, who doubted if they came closer to God or Truth in an absolute sense. Yet, they served to the last.

Why?

Probably because real service is never about what we might expect from it, even if we are expecting something like spiritual progress. We just do it because we are moved from within. It is a bit of a chicken and egg thing. Which comes first, spiritual progress or service? It can work either way.

One thing is for sure. Sincere service for others comes from within us and cannot be structured externally, at least not entirely. It is the difference between service and servitude. One we will freely choose, and the other is imposed on us, perhaps even by our own internal mental tyranny. Ironically, the danger in living by strictly enforced rules of conduct is that it can be spiritually counterproductive. Clearly, free choosing is preferred. The heart cannot be opened by holding on. Only by letting go. Then we can see that the needs of others are as important to us as our own needs, and we will be drawn to serve. It is the essence of the *Golden Rule*: "Do unto others as you would have them do unto you."

This is *right action*. Additional guidelines on right action are covered in the yoga limbs of Yama (restraints) and Niyama (observances), in Chapter 2.

Is right action cause or effect on our spiritual path? The question arises: What brings us to a point in our life where we may freely choose to do less harm, and to serve others more than we did before? Is it our rising bhakti? Is it others encouraging us to do it by their own example? Is it our daily deep meditation and its resulting inner silence?

It is all of these.

Once we find ourselves choosing to do more for others, it can become a habit, not necessarily an entirely good one in the beginning, because there will be feedback – positive reinforcement. We will be complimented for our service. We will be admired and revered. People may even give us money so we can continue to serve on an ever-larger scale. We may be tempted to continue for those reasons alone. Then what becomes of our bhakti, our chosen ideal, and the relationship of our activity to our deep meditation and other yoga practices? For those who enter service as a profession, it can become a bit muddled.

Does this mean we should not serve? No, it doesn't mean that. But we will be wise to keep our service in proportion to our inner call, particularly as it relates to our bhakti and spiritual practices.

For those who want to change the world, the advice is simple: Stand up for what you believe in, while cultivating inner silence in deep meditation each day. Consider the lives and works of great people like Gandhi, Martin Luther King and Mother Theresa of Calcutta. Move as stillness moves, not as fear would have you move.

But service is not mainly about doing great things that may draw the world's attention. Only a few are called to that. Rather, service is about what we are doing right now. It is about our present relationships and current opportunities we have to help, and taking that next step to help someone – anyone. We are lucky to have responsibilities and know people who are in need right here right now. Being able to say "yes" to that is a step on our spiritual path, as we continue to maintain balance and good self-pacing in our bhakti, practices, and daily routine of activities. As we open here and now within ourselves, we are opening the entire world.

Living a family life can draw us deeper into practices and service, leading to much joy and fulfillment. The greatest challenge that family life presents on the spiritual path is the need to provide for everyone while also making the time for practices. It takes a strong commitment, a lot of bhakti. There are many rewards if one keeps in balance.

Some may prefer to focus only on their spiritual life. This is not so simple either. Without adequate engagement in the world, renunciates can become ingrown and narrow in their outlook, with little regard for others, and stunted in their spiritual progress even while doing many yoga practices.

Service to "a family" of some kind is necessary to keep the heart and spiritual progress growing. The family may be our neighbor who needs help, our spouse and children, our community, or all of humanity. A joining that connects us to others in service is important, no matter who we are. It is an essential part of everyone's path, especially in the later stages of spiritual opening, when it is all about cultivating the divine flow in daily living – bringing the inner reality into outer manifestation.

If our path is in marriage and family life, that is great. Whether we are married or not, it is likely we will find ourselves gravitating toward a role in life that puts us in the position of having some responsibility to help someone other than ourselves.

If we are helping others, we are helping ourselves. It is the oldest wisdom in the scriptures. It will happen naturally as stillness begins to move out from us in waves of ecstatic bliss.

Real service is based in abiding inner silence, the *witness*, and is not affected by outer circumstances, or the sirens of praise or material rewards, whether they come or not. We can say that inner silence is the primary prerequisite for service that will be progressive for our own spiritual development, as well as for those who we may serve. In this sense, bhakti that calls us to daily meditation first is more fundamental to our spiritual progress than bhakti that calls us to service. If the meditation comes first, then we will surely be drawn to service that is evolutionary rather than binding.

While we may be attending to those who are in need, the real import of our service to them and to ourselves will be in the love that is conveyed relationally through our inner silence. If there is inner silence stirring, the heart will melt, and this is the essential dynamic of service. Once this process is underway, the service itself will promote the melting and increase the flow of divine love coming from within. Before inner silence is abiding, there can be doubts, and the service may be forced. We will know it when we feel it, and we should self-pace our service as necessary, like any other yoga practice.

There are many levels of service. It begins at home, wherever that happens to be and with whomever we are in relationship with on a daily basis.

Big openings come from small acts of service, when we are ready.

If we are hungry for our inner growth (cultivating bhakti) and are engaged in daily deep meditation, we will be naturally inclined to engage in service. We don't have to make a big thing of it. We can begin by doing a few more chores around the house that maybe we were not inclined to do before. We can meet the negativity we find in ourselves and in those around us with more kindness. We can forgive, which is the greatest service we can offer to anyone, and to ourselves. A heart in constant forgiveness of the ills of the world, near and far, is a heart in constant service.

The saints and sages take as much joy in the small acts of service as in the big ones. It is all the same to one who is becoming stillness in action.

The transformation does not happen overnight. As we continue along our path, desiring a closer connection with the divine within us, and engaging in deep meditation and other spiritual practices, we will see a gradual rise in our empathy for those around us. A little bit more each month and year, we will be able to forgive ourselves and others, and our conduct will slowly rise to become a natural outflow. As this happens we will have less awareness about what positive feedback may or may not be coming as a result of our positive actions. The so-called fruits of our action will matter less and less.

At the same time, we will notice any negative effects of our actions much more acutely, and be inclined to make the necessary corrections to reduce negative consequences for ourselves and others. Our actions will become increasingly intuitive. We will sense consequences before we engage in the actions that will bring them about, and act accordingly for the most positive result, even while being not much attached to the outcome. Like the great concert pianist who hears all of the notes from first to last in every moment she is playing, so too will our actions in the divine flow optimize the results.

While it is true that, ultimately, karma yoga is action without attachment to its fruits, it is also action with the most evolutionary outcome. It is a natural inner process that occurs in stillness. In time, it becomes automatic.

This kind of service begins in our ordinary life. If it expands to a broader arena, affecting many others, it will be according to our own inclinations. What we can do at home, we can do everywhere. If we are making a big reputation by serving very publicly, and are not doing so at home, then our path will be flawed. It is said that the spiritual depth of a sage is known not by the public life, but by the personal life.

The scope of our actions is influenced by karma also. There are particular inclinations each of us have, and we can follow them for the greater good. There is no such thing as "good" or "bad" karma. Only the expression of karma today in following our inclinations, which become elevated in purpose as we move forward on our spiritual path, expressed in the specific actions we take to manifest those inclinations in the present.

In other words, our present spiritual condition determines the expression of our karma. If we have a karmic tendency to be intense and impatient in performing tasks, then this may be expressed as an intensity and impatience to maximize the pace of spiritual progress in ourselves and in those around us. Of course it can be too much at times, and this is why self-pacing is advised. Yet, the karmic energy that may have otherwise gone to creating unpleasant friction in life, goes to advancing spiritual progress with the elements of bhakti and spiritual practices in the picture. There are many instances where negative experiences have inspired people to great positive accomplishments.

Like emotional energy, karma is energy that can be automatically directed by the spiritual practitioner to its highest manifestation. And in doing so, the consequences of actions undertaken become elevated.

It will happen in ordinary life, in our work, in our family, and in our interactions with everyone we may encounter. It can be as simple as just being there for a someone in need, or as complex as organizing and managing a massive aid program on the institutional level. Whatever the call may be, and whatever we choose to do within that context, inner silence will elevate the outcome in ways that are far beyond human reckoning. Like that, in advanced karma yoga, we are channels for the divine.

From this perspective, every event we encounter in life becomes an opening in pure bliss consciousness. Even as we mourn the tragedies that inevitably will visit us in life, we know that loss and adversity can lead us to new outpourings of divine love and spiritual realization. The best way to honor the past is to fully honor the present, attending to the well-being of those who are with us today. This is bhakti and karma yoga in action.

The role of service in spiritual life is both effect and cause. Service is an effect of rising inner silence, and a cause of the transformation of all karma to its most positive influence for the evolution of humanity and all of manifest existence. This is the sole purpose of karma, and its fulfillment is found in our fulfillment. Our evolution is the same as the evolution of the entire cosmos. As we undergo the process of purification and opening in our nervous system, we act accordingly. It is the gentle favoring of stillness in all action, much the same as the gentle favoring of the mantra in the simple technique of deep meditation.

From there, all we must do is go out and engage in normal daily activity, following our heart's desire, expressing toward our chosen ideal. Stillness will take care of the rest.

Chapter 4 – Passionate Living

We are all passionate about something. Our work. Our play. Our family. Our aversions. Whatever it is, we can take it to a higher plane through bhakti. It is simply a matter of investing our emotional energy in a chosen ideal that reaches beyond where we are today in terms of our life experience. Our passion can be expanding in that way.

Of course, to do this, it is necessary to look beyond where we are to what can be. It is necessary to dream a little.

Dreamers are often criticized as being impractical. But is it so impractical to imagine our greater possibilities, and move toward them? Can we ever become more if we do not have a vision, an ideal to invest ourselves in? This is true of everything we may aspire to in this life. <u>Dare to dream, and dare to act on your dream.</u>

It is the same in spiritual life, only the stakes are much higher. We can dare to dream of enlightenment in this life, and we can dare to act on that dream.

Even if we don't know quite how to dream it, we can inquire about it:

"Who am I?"

If our emotional energy is invested in the inquiry, the answers will be there to lead us along our path. It works like magic. When our sincere longing is expressed, nature will find ways to bring us grace. The act of longing with a willingness to act without too many expectations is grace itself in action.

It is a process of desire, leading to action, leading to results, leading to more desire, leading to more action, and so on...

The end result will be the union of inner divine life with outer material life. *Stillness in action.*

A Journey from Here to Here

Spiritual life is often a paradox. Sometimes the paradox is expressed in the teachings themselves. We are told to relinquish our desires, while at the same time to hunger and thirst for the divine. We are told to engage in action, even as we are advised to release our attachment to the fruits of action. We are entreated to *be in the world but not of the world.* Some may even advise us to forget about the world altogether, abiding only in the *Self.* But still we have to get up in the morning.

When these kinds of teachings are taken at face value, there can be confusion, or obsessive behavior toward one extreme or the other that can retard our spiritual progress rather than enhance it. These teachings may be accurate within the context of the lives of those who are giving them, but may not be relevant to all who are hearing or reading them. In any case, spiritual progress cannot be sustained on the basis of conceptual thinking. It is beyond ideas. Hence, the contradictions. Only in abiding inner silence can the truth be known.

Bhakti offers a big advantage in considering the paradoxes and other distractions encountered on the spiritual path, because it ignores them! Devotion is pure emotion, and does not have to puzzle things out. Little thinking is necessary.

As it says in the Bible, "Seek first the kingdom of heaven, and all will be added to you." The heart knows this.

Love knows no reason, and this enables one with strong bhakti to cut through the distractions, and <u>act</u>. If action is applied in effective spiritual practices, then the journey will be on, and the paradoxes and spiritual experiences will become a matter of record, passing scenery in the process of human spiritual transformation, rather than an endless series of evaluations. Just milestones along the road.

Road from where to where?

From *here to here*, of course. Where else would we go?

Another element of the divine paradox is the idea that we must travel far to attain enlightenment, even while there is nowhere to go. Another way of putting it is to say that there is much to do, yet nothing to do. As with other spiritual paradoxes, if *doing without doing* is intellectualized too much, we may find extreme behavior emerging. Like the person who leaves life's responsibilities, spouse and children, running off to seek enlightenment. Or the seeker who discontinues all activity in the belief that there is nothing to do, thus becoming a burden on those around them.

Whether the aspirant runs away or sits down and does nothing, the essential fact will not be changed. That is, we take ourselves wherever we go. So no matter where we go or what we do or not do, the journey will be from here to here – from not realizing to realizing our ever-present *Self.*

We don't have to leave our home or disengage from our responsibilities to reach this realization. All we must do is long for it, spend some time each day in structured practices like deep meditation and spinal breathing pranayama, and then go out and live our life normally. With that, we will be traveling quickly on the inside in purification and opening, without doing much out of the ordinary on the outside. We don't have to put on strange clothing, take up a new lifestyle, or engage in elaborate rituals. We can do these things if we are strongly drawn to them, but it will only make a difference if it inspires us internally in some way. The same thing can be accomplished in jeans and a T-shirt, sitting where we are right now.

While enlightenment is ultimately a non-doing, a letting go, we must do something to cultivate it.

We can wait for someone else to turn on the light (maybe a very long time), or we can get up and turn on the light ourselves. We must do something in order to do nothing. And we do not have to leave home to do it.

In fairness to the old ways, things are quite different now. Information about the means and processes of human spiritual transformation are readily available these days. It is the information age, and nearly everyone has access to knowledge. In the old days, one might have to travel far to find knowledge. And the knowledge often had strings attached – required lifestyle, beliefs, rituals, etc. Even so, the journey has always been within each person, and it will always be like that. Now, with greatly increased access to spiritual information, we can move beyond the external props of spiritual life, and boil it down to the basic principles and methods, which are universal. What we find is an endless expanding cycle of spiritual desire, action, purification and opening, continuing on until enlightenment and the paradoxes of spirit become part of everyday life and are little noticed.

Along the way, we will have many experiences. We may feel extremely passionate about our spiritual journey in the beginning, even before we have traveled very far. In practicing daily deep meditation over months and years, we will come to know inner silence and reside in *That*, finding it to be our own

Self. Ordinary life will go on, even as we find ourselves living beyond it, untouched by it. We will find the rise of dispassion amidst the normal passions of living. We might wonder if we are losing it, with respect to being engaged in life.

As we continue on, we will find that our desire has not been dissolved, but transformed. Transformed from personal desire to divine desire. This is the gradual shift from serving self (our body/mind) to serving *Self* found everywhere around us in others. During this transformation, we will find our attachment to the outcomes of all action becoming less.

It has been said that desire leads to action, and to attachment to the results of the action. Yet, as we move forward on our spiritual path, we find that our desire shifts to become more for the action itself – the divine flow coming through us – and not so much for the end result. The desire and divine flow become one. In becoming one like that, our actions become a powerful force of evolution in all that we do in our everyday life. It is the power of love – outpouring divine love.

We find ourselves living a passionate life with dispassion, a life filled with desires without expectations, and a life of full engagement in active surrender. This is possible through ongoing devotion and the rise of inner silence.

Our initial spiritual desire continues throughout our journey and transforms gradually from personal to divine. We have gone nowhere, except forward in the realization of our own *Self* – a journey from here to here. We have become love on the move, stillness in action, which is the marriage of stillness and divine ecstasy radiating constantly from within us. Then all of life becomes our *divine beloved* and all we do is a glorious dance unfolding unity everywhere. The journey begins in love, and ends in love.

The Dance of Unity

There is a misconception that enlightenment is about doing nothing. We are told to stop thinking, stop desiring, stop doing. A practical person might get the impression that enlightenment is very impractical. After all, if the journey is about stopping everything, why be born in the first place? The world isn't such a bad place, and in being here we have the rare opportunity to make it better. So, why renounce the world? The world and we are all one thing anyway, the great cosmic *Self*. So what is there to renounce? A more flexible approach to enlightenment is found in the advice to *serve God* or *Truth*. The Zen Buddhists take a less dramatic approach, boiling it down to *chop wood, carry water*.

In other words, undergo the process of human spiritual transformation while doing something, and then continue doing something according to need. The doing will then be all the better for everyone, including ourselves. This is the fruit of bhakti and karma yoga.

Enlightenment without action is like an egg with no chicken. It is mere potential without expression, which is what we all are *before* enlightenment. Therefore enlightenment without action, without outer expressions, isn't enlightenment at all. Be wary of teachings that promote non-doing. In our heart we will know it is not complete.

There can be no divine union until there is engagement – action. The one who is enlightened will be more active than ever before, because they will be engaged everywhere on every level, visible and invisible. And all the while they will be doing nothing at all – *stillness in action*. There is that paradox again. Don't mind it. Just keep going in bhakti and practices and you will see for yourself what it is. So when the sages tell us that enlightenment is non-doing, what they mean is *non-doing in doing*.

Bhakti without action is like a car without wheels. The engine may turn and make lots of noise, but the car is going nowhere. It is similar to self-inquiry with limited inner silence, which we call *non-relational*. Lots of movement in the mind, but little traction in stillness. The heart needs objects to love and interact with just as the mind needs abiding inner silence to express itself in ways that are in *relationship* with the truth within us. Take away one side of either equation, and there will be imbalance, which is often expressed in some sort of extremism. When we see an extremist, we can immediately see that the equation is not balanced. This is why integrated multi-pronged paths of practice are much more effective and joyful than obsessive single-pronged approaches.

The path to union is a joining of two dynamics within and around us – a divine romance intimately associated with our bhakti.

Over time, we can readily observe the two poles joining in our neurobiology and emotional and mental functioning:

- **Stillness** – A natural slowdown in metabolism, and rise of a silent inner observer, the witness.

- **Ecstasy** – A radiance occurring in the nervous system, illuminating the whole body, and beyond.

Even as we are becoming untouched by events in time, space and materiality, we are also becoming passionate as we directly experience the ecstatic nature of life within and around us. As our mind comes to be observed as a natural fluctuation in a infinite pool of stillness, our heart comes to be known as an ever-expanding radiation of love. These two dynamics merge within us and radiate outward as stillness in action, ecstatic bliss and outpouring divine love. Our actions are colored accordingly. The result is service to God and Truth, even as we are chopping the wood and carrying the water of everyday life. It is life lived as spectacular and ordinary at the same time. *Spectacular ordinariness*. It has also been called living in a state of *grace*.

But really, it is only life lived the way it can be lived by all of us, and it will be, because we are all wired for it. It is the destiny of the human race. This is much more than an individual dynamic. It is a dynamic that encompasses all of us. What happens in anyone is happening in everyone. Ultimately we all rise or fall together. Fortunately, we are on the rise. It is the natural course of evolution occurring.

Human spiritual transformation is as natural and inevitable as the lowly caterpillar becoming the beautiful butterfly fluttering away on the breeze. It isn't for a few of us. It is for all of us. It is not something that is done to us. It is something we do for ourselves, because we all contain the seed of enlightenment. This is certain, and it has been proclaimed by the wise since the dawn of humanity.

Actively surrendering each day to our spiritual transformation is to become the divine, which is our essential nature. It is a gradual development. It does not happen in one day. It goes by degrees. First we surrender to the ideal of becoming more – maybe just to the question, "Who am I, and why am I here?" With this thread of surrender we can be inspired to begin daily practice of deep meditation. Then, with some inner silence coming up, we can surrender to adding spinal breathing pranayama. Then this can lead to other practices, etc. At some point, divine ecstasy rises in us, conducted simultaneously and permanently throughout our body, and then we become sold out to the beautiful ecstatic energies (kundalini) transforming us from within. Total surrender comes step-by-step with our advancing experiences. To have advancing experiences we need to be doing daily practices. So surrender and daily practice go hand in hand. This is why the role of desire becoming devotion to our expanding chosen ideal is discussed throughout the AYP writings. We cultivate direct experience every step along the way, and surrender comes along with it through the natural interconnectedness of the limbs of yoga.

Eventually our experience rises to the level of unshakable inner silence, ecstatic bliss and outpouring divine love. By then we have become that which we have been surrendering to. Total surrender is enlightenment. It is immutable, beyond all affirmations and strategies of the mind. Total surrender is a heart constantly overflowing.

Now it is time for us to claim our destiny like never before. We can do so simply by allowing our innermost longing for wholeness to find expression in practical spiritual methods that will hasten the purification and opening that is occurring in us in this moment. It is always happening in us. All we need to do is tap into it, and it will accelerate.

With our rising bhakti and willingness to act, it is a joyful dance we are inviting ourselves to. The dance of unity. The more we open and the more we flow from within, the more will unity be expressing in the awareness of everyone. The momentum of spirit is real, as anyone who is engaged on their path knows. It is not fantasy. We can feel it within ourselves in the form of inner silence and ecstatic conductivity, and we can see it occurring in the flow of events in our life.

The more we long for it, and the more we act, the more joyful and unifying the dance becomes.

Our thoughts, feelings and actions will flow naturally from within, and the mystery will dissolve. Life becomes a celebration of divine love, dancing in the *One*...

Further Reading and Support

Yogani is an American spiritual scientist who, for more than thirty years, has been integrating ancient techniques from around the world which cultivate human spiritual transformation. The approach he has developed is non-sectarian, and open to all. In the order published, his books include:

Advanced Yoga Practices – Easy Lessons for Ecstatic Living
A large user-friendly textbook providing 240 detailed lessons on the AYP integrated system of yoga practices.

The Secrets of Wilder – A Novel
The story of young Americans discovering and utilizing actual secret practices leading to human spiritual transformation.

The AYP Enlightenment Series
Easy-to-read instruction books on yoga practices, including:

- *Deep Meditation – Pathway to Personal Freedom*
- *Spinal Breathing Pranayama – Journey to Inner Space*
- *Tantra – Discovering the Power of Pre-Orgasmic Sex*
- *Asanas, Mudras and Bandhas – Awakening Ecstatic Kundalini*
- *Samyama – Cultivating Stillness in Action, Siddhis and Miracles*
- *Diet, Shatkarmas and Amaroli – Yogic Nutrition and Cleansing for Health and Spirit*
- *Self Inquiry – Dawn of the Witness and the End of Suffering*
- *Bhakti and Karma Yoga – The Science of Devotion and Liberation Through Action*
- *Eight Limbs of Yoga – The Structure and Pacing of Self-Directed Spiritual Practice*

For up-to-date information on the writings of Yogani, and for the free *AYP Support Forums*, please visit:

www.advancedyogapractices.com

CPSIA information can be obtained at www.ICGtesting.com
Printed in the USA
BVOW04s1739180514

353494BV00016B/603/P